"Thank you for the fantastic support you gave me to help my husband heal and get well. I appreciate your insight and spiritual strength."
Kim B.

"All these natural products and methods can sure be confusing, thanks for being someone I can talk to about it and get experience and knowledge from."
Tamara A.

"I was so inspired to read on OXYGEN/LYME. Mostly inspired as you are a mother and have children recovering. Your story appears to be like mine as far as passing it too children during pregnancy. I will continue to read your blog.
Monique B.

1

Surviving Lyme

Janice Fairbairn

To the many prayer warriors who through their prayers, help guide our family to healing. To the many Lymies and "healthnuts" we have met along our journey that introduced us to a better lifestyle and to these methods of healing.

To my heartfriends, Nan, Amy, Rose Marie and Lisha. Thank you for wiping my tears, making me laugh and praying me to success.

To my doctors, Dr. Jernigan, Dr. Cox, and Dr. Jowdy, thank you for being vessels for God's healing power and knowledge and for dedicating your lives to healing in His will.

I remain confident of this:
I will see the goodness of the LORD
in the land of the living.

Wait for the LORD;
be strong and take heart
and wait for the LORD.

(Psalm 27:13-14)

Table of Contents

Before You Begin – Symptom List

Before we even begin to discuss Lyme, let's create a baseline in your life. Put checkmarks in the lines next to the following lists of symptoms and autoimmune disorders. After you have done your checkmarks, if you have doubts about your children or someone else you know, make checkmarks in a different color for them. How many did you get? Enough to be certain or to make you want to get tested?

Almost all of the dozens of people I've met getting treated for Lyme had been diagnosed with one or more autoimmune disorders. I had been diagnosed with four. Everyone I met had thyroid problems or an autoimmune disorder of the thyroid, most had either hearing or sight problems and many had some sort of neurological issue, like tingling, numbness, twitching, etc.

Lyme disease and the neurotoxins it produces in its life cycle are deadly and cause havoc on the immune system causing it to misfire and attack anything around that moves (or so it seems).

There is no hard and fast rule to how many of these symptoms you check "yes" to have Lyme disease. I can only tell you that it seems to me that most people with at least one autoimmune disorder, thyroid problems, low body temperature and increased allergies or allergic reactions should think seriously about getting tested or beginning treatment.

All of the following symptoms are possible and have been recorded with Lyme disease and its co-infections.

Chart of Symptoms for Lyme

http://www.lymeresearchalliance.org/signs-symptom-list.html

Also consider the following Autoimmune Disorders as signs that the underlying cause could be Lyme:

- Acute Coronary Syndrome
- Fibromyalgia
- Chronic Fatigue Syndrome
- Hashimoto's Hypothyroidism
- Graves' Disease/Hyperthyroidism
- Rheumatoid Arthritis
- Krohns Disease
- Irritable Bowel Syndrome
- Sjogren's Syndrome
- Parkinsons'
- Multiple Sclerosis
- Alzheimer's
- Dimentia
- Lupus
- Depression
- Autism
- ADHD

- Aspergers
- Dyslexia
- Psychological Disorders – Obsessive Compulsive, etc.
- Meniere's
- TMJ
- Celiac
- Addison's Disease
- Diabetes
- Cushing's Disease
- Polycystic Ovary Syndrome
- Restless Leg Syndrome
- Schizophrenia

Introduction

How did it start for me? Well, I had a miscarriage, two difficult deliveries, early onset para-menopause and borderline glaucoma. Soon after kids, I began to get some more hormone swinging and "anger" that was driving me crazy. Both my kids had severe digestion and behavior issues. My son would have been diagnosed Asperger's and we were losing him farther down the spectrum before we began to do more health changes. My daughter had asthma, speech delays, hearing, emotional and sleep disturbances. My life was a constant duct-taped stress ball. Held barely together at the seams, it felt like the person at the circus trying to keep all the plates spinning in the air. Those plates crashing down became a fear I lived with daily.

Thanks to the kid's health issues, our household got healthier and healthier. We were eating all organic, gluten free, casein free and soy free. We bought only organic or grass fed meats. My husband and I began to do 10 day fast/cleanses at the beginning of every year. It was at this point that we began to notice my hormone swings got worse.

I had been going to our chiropractor/kinesiologist for years and he had been guiding my supplements and health regiment to try to clear out toxic estrogen, etc. It helped but didn't help.

I finally sought out the counsel of a trusted Naturopath doctor in Kansas City that helped us so much with my son's Asperger's. After doing countless tests, he discovered I had no adrenal function, my cholesterol was through the roof, and my hormones were leaning into menopause (at 39). No wonder I was a mess. He began a natural regiment to address these issues. It included some cortisol supplements, methylation support, progesterone, and cat's claw for the cholesterol.

After the first few months my test showed huge improvement. Cholesterol way down, energy up, hormones more in balance. I felt better. At the time, I should have noticed, but it didn't register. I began to have some chest tightness and pain that radiated from the center of my chest. Over the next few months, I continued the regiment. The chest pain heightened. Due to life and busyness, I cast it aside, not wanting to deal with one more symptom of something. My husband started his own business the year before and life was at a new level of nuts.

Finally, I realized late one night as I couldn't sleep because the chest pain was so severe, that I had to do something about it. Dreams of lung cancer (I was an ex-smoker) or heart attack raced through my mind. I also had surgery on my esophagus in college to remove tissue webbing and it was very close to that area of my sternum.

A few weeks later, we went for a family walk one afternoon and I got severe chest constriction, pain and dizziness and almost passed out. My vision got "weird" and my heart rate wasn't recovering. So we went to the ER and had every test run in the book and they released me as fine. I then followed up with a regular doctor. I called the ND in Kansas City and told him what happened. We stopped the protocol for a few weeks just in case, took blood tests and then began to ease them back in one at a time.

Bam! Again, this time worse, extreme nausea. I began to react to foods I was eating that I had never had problems with before. I quickly lost 10 lbs. (starting at 115). I began to supplement my diet with medical food shakes and super greens. I had to stop the super greens, because they would make the nausea and dizziness intensify.

That began a 3 month journey through traditional medicine and its ability to try to determine what on earth was going on. CT scans, MRI (to rule out brain tumor), Gastrointestinal tests to rule out celiac, Pylori, etc. Two esophageal scopes to rule out return of the tissue webbing. Nope. Nothing wrong with me – take an anti-nausea and an anti-depressant. None of the anti-nausea at any dose made a dent in the nausea. I never would take the anti-depressants. I was frustrated, sick, in pain, but not depressed.

Sicker and sicker I became. There was more and more weight loss, no sleep, immense pain in chest, heart and under ribcage. I couldn't drive, couldn't read, and I felt like I was going blind. Intermittently while seeing the other doctors; I was also seeing my eye doctor often to try to pinpoint what was going on with my failing and erratic vision.

I had been diagnosed Sjogren's, Lupus, Hashimoto's, Glaucoma and other possible autoimmune diseases. Why? I had never been healthier. We had no familial history of autoimmune, except for my older sister with Hashimoto's. I had learned a lot about autoimmune with my son's ASD. I knew the body was being attacked by something that causes the immune system to dysfunction and attack itself; hence the autoimmune. But now what?

I had the doctors run every urine/stool panel they could, looking for critters – parasites/viruses/bacteria and all came back clear. Impossible. There had to be something triggering my immune system. I had read lots of books about oxygen therapy from my dad. Ok, I decided. I will boost my immune system by pushing into it pure oxygen through intravenous Ozone treatments. Take that whatever critter is in there flying under the radar. I'll get you somehow. (see resources section)

I called an "outside the box" MD I knew and scheduled IV ozone therapy. I called there for an appointment because I needed someone to look at my problems, my health issues from an entirely different perspective. I knew this doctor wouldn't think pharmaceutical quick fix, but would actually listen and try to find the root cause of the problem. The first oxygen therapy session was awesome; I hadn't felt better in months. That's it; I just needed to help the immune system fight off whatever it was. I did another one three days later and Bam. Another crash. The worst one yet.

That crash lasted three days before it faded out. The crashes became filled with more and more symptoms; dizziness, extreme nausea, sleepy but restless, horrific pain under my ribcage, chest constriction, dry mouth, hands and feet numb and tingling, tightness and pain in chest, headaches, and hot tingling pain in head and temples. After that recovery, my dad (nutritionist) agreed with the theory that the immune system needed a boost and to try colloidal silver instead of the oxygen. By the third dose. Crash. Bad crash.

Why better and then worse. What was causing the crashes? I met with this "outside the box" MD again and spent 10 minutes giving him the lowdown. His response was simple. Get tested for Lyme. What, Lyme? Yes, it could cause all this.

Went back to my family regular doctor and begged and had to threaten to get tested for Lyme. He agreed reluctantly and I got a positive on the Western Blot and the DNA PCR test. Both doctors recommended I begin Doxycycline for three weeks right away. The "outside the box" doctor suggested I keep doing the Ozone with the Doxy to support the immune system and add in some liver support for the detoxing.

At this point I was probably 95 lbs. and very weak and exhausted emotionally and physically. I had already been up and down for almost 5 months. But we had our answer and it would be over soon. People get this all the time, right? They just take antibiotics and live life. Wrong.

This began the darkest days I have ever experienced and I wouldn't wish upon my worst enemy. What I didn't know at the time was that what I had been experiencing was herxing. Severe herxing. Some that caused us to go the ER again and again. The worst had me in full body tremors/seizures. They released me each time with "nothing wrong" and "give her antidepressants and something to help her sleep".

I did the Doxy and stopped the ozone because I literally couldn't handle both. I was taking liver support but still felt so sick and nauseous it pales in comparison to how sick I felt before. I could eat nothing. I was only drinking the medical food shakes and water. And that was a battle. I couldn't leave the house – everything and everywhere we went gave my severe migraines, dizziness and vertigo.

It was at the end of this three weeks that I finally looked at my husband and said call the church and ask for prayer. I just knew I was going to die. Down to below 85 lbs. and unable to eat and the pain was unbearable. In the meantime I was having my dad or husband scour the internet for a place I could go and be checked in and do Lyme treatment. I was desperate. I knew without a handout in this pit, an absolute miracle, it would be the end of me. I had called the doctor to tell them how bad I felt and I had been to the ER and no one seemed to care that I was disappearing.

After the prayers went out, three days in a row by three different people I was handed a Lyme doctor's name. Then another two people gave me a different Lyme doctor's name out of state. One in Missouri and one right here in Wichita, KS. I called to make appointments, not sure how I was going to make the trip to MO, but realized I needed to see someone who knew more about Lyme and herxing. I got cancellation appointments the following week and the Wichita, KS doctor was first and it ended up being the place we chose and didn't even go to MO.

19

What I didn't know then that I know now was that the neurotoxin and ammonia overload from the Cat's Claw, the Ozone, the Colloidal Silver and finally the Doxy had flooded my system in trying to kill off the Lyme and co-infections. I was herxing myself right to the grave. My brain and heart were filled with ammonia, my gall bladder, liver and kidneys were 80% non-functioning. My lymph system was a clogged up solidified mess and my blood was not only thick and lifeless, but not flowing out of my brain due to jugular blocks from the Lyme bacteria.

I was as good as dead. In that health condition, I bet I wouldn't have lasted more than a few weeks. God had other plans.

The Lyme doctors I chose do a holistic approach with NO antibiotics. They also do not believe in herxing. In fact, over the course of my treatment, I only experienced the beginnings of two more herxing episodes that they put a stop to almost immediately. I am not kidding. I am so serious. I fought off and and am Lyme free without herxing. I know it sounds unbelievable but it is true. I did not believe them either. I thought, sure, they are just going to try to drug me to make me forget I am herxing.

I mean I had been in a herx for nearly four weeks straight without a break. The other ones had come in three to ten days waves and usually dissipated a bit. This one had come in to camp and hadn't left. I was so thin that I had to use a butt pillow to sit on most of the chairs in our house. I was so exhausted I could hardly get up out of bed each day and make it down the stairs.

The doctors there at Hansa Center of Optimum Health, the founder a former Lymie, developed this protocol to save his own life, antibiotic free. All three doctors have experienced Lyme so they get it. They believe in detoxing the ammonia and neurotoxins as a top priority in order to then strengthen your body to fight off the Lyme itself, as it was designed to do. (see Resources section)

They used bio-resonance testing and found I had the trifecta of Lyme (borrelia, babesia and bartonellis), Rocky Mountain Spotted Fever, West Nile Virus, mycoplasma, parasites and just about any and every pathogen out there were all invited to the party going on in my body. The oddest thing they told me and it took weeks before I could actually cognitively process the information: that I had a condition called CCSVI.

CCSVI standing for Chronic Cerebrospinal Venous Insufficiency means that the Lyme bacteria has caused closures in the jugular veins coming out of my brain so the blood flowing into the brain has no place to flow out. My left side almost completely closed off and the right side about halfway. So what happens to the blood being pumped into the brain if it has no way out? Well, it causes tremendous pressure and iron buildup in the tissue and flows backward down the arteries. Upriver so to speak. It is called back flowing. It causes erratic heart beats, severe chest pressure and pain, brain fog and memory loss.

I chose to tell you all this so you know I have walked into the deepest part of the valley where you are or where you have been. I have met people who suffered more and less. I have met three generations in one family all suffering all the way down to the eight year old. I have met entire households struck with this terrible illness and all fighting for their lives. I get passionate; I get fired up at the lack of support from the traditional medical community and how hard you have to fight to get traction in this illness. I get frustrated on how much money it costs to pay all these treatments out of pocket because there is no alternative in traditional medicine. If there was enough time in each day I would talk to each of you personally and coach, pray and encourage you through this process because, believe me, we all need the support. If there was enough money on our money tree, I would give it all to people desperate to get natural treatment but can't afford it.

There is so much misinformation out there and not enough good information. It feels like the brain fog I had was passed by osmosis to each Allopathic doctor to keep me shrouded in misery. They are not helping us!!

Now as I look back on my path and process, there are of course, some things I would do differently. If you are reading this because you are aware of something but don't know what it is for sure or haven't launched your official attack on Lyme yet, or have had failed attempts with antibiotics – here is my updated list of what I would do. This by no means covers everything, but gives you a place to start, a place to launch your initial attack for successfully and to have the endurance to finish the race strong.

Warning:

Before you begin to read the remainder of this book, let me strongly caution you as to how to apply it in your life. Do not sit at home by yourself and try to kill this Lyme disease off in your body by using some of these methods. **Do not try this at home alone.** *This Lyme thing is mean and tough and will not leave willingly without a fight. Use this information as a framework and knowledge base as to how you are going to launch a war against this Lyme in your life. Use it to provoke questions and new treatments with your doctor or team of doctors. Since I am not a qualified doctor, none of these recommendations come with a guarantee or without negative consequences.*

Section 1 - Find the Right Doctor

I would find the best, most qualified Lyme doctor using natural treatments I can find. I would then find a local doctor of natural bent that could support this long distance treatment and that I could use for quick short term checkups. Building this team is crucial. Absolutely crucial. Both these doctors need to understand detoxification and how Lyme works. If they don't know about neurotoxins and ammonia damage and Post Lyme Syndrome and herxing then RUN FOR THE DOOR.

Interview different doctors and have them lay out their protocol recommendation for you or your loved one. Compare and contrast their protocols then go back and ask questions about the discrepancies to fully understand where they are coming from. Be sure about their comprehension of the human body and the Lyme. Ask them for testimonials and success rate. When you are in the lobby of each doctor's office (every time) make friends. I introduce myself to everyone who comes into the lobby of my doctor and I talk to them, really talk to them. You don't know me so you don't know how hard this is for me because I'm not a "love talking to strangers" kind of person. It is critical for you to know the success rate and treatment protocol of other patients and if they are feeling better. Later, I realized I must keep up the "talking to everybody phenomenon" because the newbies, like I was, need to hear about success and that they picked the right place. It is incredibly encouraging to hear from patients "this place is healing me". We are on this journey to encourage one another.

The husband of a friend of mine has some horrible form of cancer that I cannot pronounce and she said the traditional cancer program is depressing. No one in the program is getting better and she sees death everywhere they go and every time they are there. SCARY! I would run for the hills. Every program is not for everyone, but the wellness numbers should safely be in the 80% and 90% to be sure the doctors know what they are doing.

The bad news I have to break to you before we even get into this fight, is that you will not find cooperation from your health insurance carrier in the battle. Finding even a traditional MD that insurance will cover all the treatments and services is rare. It sucks, but I have to be honest with you so you are not caught off balance and surprised. Almost all of us are paying cash or going in debt to get through this thing. To the insurance company's defense (I have no idea why I'm defending their position) most of these treatments against Lyme are ground breaking and have only been used for a few years. Anything that new, they are scared to death over providing funding for.

Just accept this fact and be delightfully surprised if yours will pay anything: Insurance will not cover this. Insurance will not cover most of these treatments. Insurance is built around traditional medicine and unless you find an M.D. who can code things in a gray area, your insurance is going to buck. If it's not a pill and it's not administered in a hospital, then good luck.

Section 2- What Kind of Doctor Am I Looking For?

My best recommendation would be to find a doctor using muscle testing, kinesiology, or bio-resonance scanning to test for Lyme and other pathogens. (see resource list) It is the only fail proof method for determining what you have and what is going on. See if there is a local Lyme support group in your area or go to chat rooms online and see who is talking about what and who. I got 4 positive and 1 negative about the doctors I chose from local testimonials. Ask around but use your discernment in what you read online. One poison apple can ruin the whole bushel. Don't forget that. I would also not be afraid to take that one negative testimonial in to the doctor and ask them to explain it.

If someone has a bad experience with a natural doctor, it is 100 times worse than with a regular doctor. Our culture has higher expectations of a doctor healing outside the box. When it does not fit or work as fast as a duct tape pharmaceutical, then we label them a failure and tell the whole world and never give anyone else in natural medicine a chance. Watch out for the 'cry wolf' testimonies and for joining in with them or listening too closely. Twelve doctors in traditional medicine failed me and were letting me die, yet, if my child breaks his arm, where am I going to go? To the ER or Emergency Clinic to get it set and cast. Those 12 doctors have not hindered my ability to discern within the industry.

I know people who have been fighting "mystery" illnesses for decades and have tried dozens of doctors and dozens of treatments yet they don't berate each of the doctors for failing. They are frustrated with the illness that none of them can find, but don't blame any of those doctors for failing. They keep going back and going back to traditional medicine to keep trying. Equally, we should allow natural medicine an opportunity. If you find one naturally trained or out of the box doctor that doesn't float your boat. Look for another. Do not write off the entire industry because of an ego, lack of knowledge or not a good fit. We all sin and fall short. Everyone you find is not going to be perfect and they will make mistakes.

Most importantly, make sure the doctor is listening, truly listening. Not just lumping you in with the masses and treating you like everyone else. Each body is different and unique and will fight the same pathogen completely different. Each of your symptoms is important and part of the code your body is using to ask for help.

If you are not familiar with these types of muscle testing doctors, you are not in the minority. The best way I can describe it is by using an analogy of "Divining for Water". The reason in the old days that certain people could use a stick and divine for water, was they were picking up on a change in frequency in the stick. God made everything in creation with a particular energy setting. Science has confirmed this, so I'm not making this up. Colors have frequency, sound has frequency, objects omit frequency. Each of these frequencies is unique. But pinecones resonate the same frequency whether you are in the US or Australia (do they have pinecones there?) Water emits the same frequency. So the trained water diviners could tell when they got close to a shallow water table by "reading" the frequency of the stick. (Read Energy Medicine by JL Oshman 2000)

Similarly, these types of doctors use frequency to "read" distress in your liver, heart, digestion, etc. A regular functioning liver should resonate a certain way. The pathogens that cause the problem also emit a particular frequency and can be found and eradicated.

Too many laboratories are failing in finding the critters in the bloodstream, urine or stool samples. If you read studies and believe in conspiracy theories, then you will understand why the labs are not "supposed" to find too many pathogens. Or why they do not do a thorough job

31

testing the samples to find pathogens. The lab that do the best job is IGenX.

Another thing to research in your area is a testing technique called the Computerized Regulated Thermography (CRT), a German technology. CRT is an FDA approved, objective and non-invasive way of evaluating your body's functions. It is the EKG of the natural physician. CRT represents one of several objective diagnostic evaluations in Integrative Medicine. It is a medical imaging method that supplies information as meaningful as MRI and X-ray, and is safe and non-invasive. Over 1500 physicians in Europe use CRT. Thermography has over 12,000 citations and studies held within current medical journals.

This particular device evaluates your body functions by a direct temperature measurement probe instead of measuring thermal radiation. The result is a scanning method that is much more precise than any other thermo graphic system. It maps out the complete autonomic nervous system as it projects to and from each organ or tissue. With this form of thermography, we can finally see what the body is doing long before it becomes dysfunctional enough to create an irreversible problem. This is not diagnosing disease, but rather identifying the patterns that lead to disease, so that these patterns can be successfully treated.

It actually detects breast cancer 7 years before a mammogram (in studies) because it detects the malfunction at the cellular level. It is instrumental in helping develop a proper healing protocol for anyone with a chronic illness. Many times, the organs in the most distress get the attention first and because the squeaky wheel gets the grease, other organs or systems go untreated just because they don't redline on a blood test. The CRT will find it. To a well-trained physician in reading the test, it can also find CCSVI without a MRI. (See Christiane-Northrup, MD on Huffington Post, The Best Breast Test: The Promise of Thermography, Oct 2010)

If you are unable to find a doctor of this type that suits you I would definitely go with a Naturopath with experience in Lyme disease. NDs tend to look at the entire body as a whole and not treat the symptoms and chase rabbit trails. They are educated to understand nutrition, diet, acupuncture or acupressure and some even cross train into chiropractic because of how the structure of the body is so closely linked to disease.

In your doctor team arsenal should be also an Lyme Literate Medical Doctor (LLMD). There aren't very many of these doctors across the country, but that number is growing. They are well versed at healing and treating Lyme and its co-infections. The only problem I have with this group is that they are still attacking Lyme with traditional methods of antibiotics. If you are like me and many others I have met that the antibiotics don't work or nearly kill them, then what choice do you have? For those who can tolerate the antibiotics, insurance is more likely to pick up the tab for a portion of this treatment. If this is your route, then find a LLMD who uses non-traditional therapies to support the body with the antibiotics.

Section 3- Detoxification

Begin a serious methylation and detoxification support protocol. Supplements, lymph massage, liver detox, colon cleanse, etc. The body has to detox what the Lyme is producing before it can be strong enough to fight it. Because in fighting it, the Lyme produces even more ammonia and it can be deadly. There are many methods out there, my favorites are detox baths, Neuro-antitox (from Jernigan Neutraceuticals), Charcoal, Sillymarin, MolyB, TMG, B12, Folic Acid, super greens like King Chorella.

Doing a blood panel and finding the weaknesses in your body's ability to detox would be a good starting place. A worthy doctor will find the holes and plug them before starting to push for more detoxing. Trying to detox before working the holes will just cause additional disruption and back up in the systems. Also finding what organs are housing the highest levels of toxins, so to know where to concentrate the organ support first.

Lymph massages or lymph treatments are similarly important in the detox process. The lymph fluid can be almost solidified in Lyme disease and extreme chronic illnesses and it is crucial to "break it up" and let the body regenerate it. Certain doctors use forms of vibration therapy to help move it along and some just recommend massage.

Far infrared saunas are likewise an incredible tool for detoxing and for killing off Lyme. I never used these because my weight and hydration were in critical conditions, but know many who have and who now own one in their homes.

Caution: do not do far infrared saunas without doctor supervision because the Lyme usually lowers the body temperature to create an environment in which it can thrive. Using detox baths and saunas is great for detoxing and healing, but can also cause the body to rise in temperature and kill off some of the Lyme in great numbers and cause major herxing.

Go in gently, gradually and let your body get used to the treatment and handle the die off and detoxing slowly. We do plan on buying one of these saunas in the near future for life long detoxing success for our family.

Many other therapies and treatments that promote detox exist and are very successful. Make sure your doctor can explain how the therapy works and how they play into your protocol and symptoms. Ask about frequency and if there are less expensive home versions available – there always are.

Water, water and more water. Make sure your body is hydrated and is hydrating. Mine wasn't doing either. They had to work hard for the first month just to get my body to accept hydration. My muscles and organs were atrophied and had to be coaxed into re-hydrating. Painful massages and other therapies were involved, but necessary to get the water in there and get it to do the healing work it can do all on its own. A well hydrated body is less likely to get chronic. I spent weeks and months drinking almost a gallon of water each day. That might sound extreme to you, but you would not believe the difference it gives your tissues in fighting infection.

Finally, talk to your doctor about a colon cleanse or detox cleanse diet. Depending on what organ is struggling or what pathogen you are fighting in your gut, let your doctor guide you into a detox or cleanse. Whether it is 7, 10, 21, or 30 days, this can jump start your body's healing. We adopted the detox/cleanse philosophy of doing one each January to cleanse out the holiday eating and begin a new year fresh. Do not just jump into one of these without "supervision" depending on how sick you are. Pushing your body too hard too fast can be damaging to your organs and filtering systems. There are supplements and medical food powders that can be used in conjunction with the diet to "assist" the body in detoxing so the release of the toxins does not get clogged up somewhere else.

The last thing you want to do is to begin a detox regiment and not drink enough water or use detox support supplements. If you do, then you could release the toxins from the liver and they end up in the colon. It is incredibly important to drink plenty of water and support the body in completely ridding the toxins all the way out.

Section 4- Oxygen Therapy

Oxygen therapy done correctly with the detox and organ support would be awesome. If I wasn't claustrophobic, I would have done hyperbaric oxygen treatments which does the most for the ammonia release from the brain. See the resource page for book titles on using oxygen either intravenously, by hyperbaric chamber or by using hydrogen peroxide in its various forms and ways.

Oxygen is a life force. We need it for survival for breathing and we are made of it, 62% to 71%. Our bodies were also designed to need it systematically. In an oxygen rich environment, the body will kill viruses, harmful bacteria, toxins, pathogens, and disease microorganisms while contributing to the vitality of healthy cells. (From The One Minute Cure by Madison Cavanaugh)

Since the 1950s oxygen has been tested and used to heal and restore function for people with various neurological disorders and injuries including:

- Alzheimer's Disease
- Parkinson's Disease
- Stroke
- Multiple Sclerosis
- Lou Gehrig's Disease (ALS)

- Brain Injury

- Learning Disability

- Cerebral Palsy

- Chronic Fatigue Syndrome

- Autism

- Lyme

In studies, cancer has also been shown to shrink in an oxygen rich environment. Oxygen therapy done correctly with the detox and organ support can be a crucial piece in healing Lyme. Disease just seeks to and thrives in an oxygen deprived environment.

In his book Alkalize or Die, Theodore Broody examines the body's healing balance from an alkaline perspective. Our bodies are in a constant state of either acidity or alkalinity. If we become to acidic, disease will thrive. Eating processed food and too much sugar and starch can do this creating an environment rich for any pathogen or disease to take hold and thrive.

To treat with oxygen, there are a variety of choices available. Store bought hydrogen peroxide can kill warts and when used in conjunction with Epsom salt in a bath, can oxygenate the body through the skin. Food grade hydrogen peroxide, when administered safely and properly can boost that healing even farther. Some doctors do ozone or peroxide intravenously to speed up the introduction directly into the bloodstream.

We frequently still use detox baths with equal parts 3% store bought hydrogen peroxide and Epsom salts for detoxing and boosting immune systems. 2-4 cups for adults (I use 2 cups for my 110lbs and my husband uses 4 cups for his 170 lbs.) We typically use 1 cup each for the kids who are around 50lbs. I have read about people who have rigged their hot tubs to be hydrogen peroxide to clean instead of chlorine and then use them for detoxification.

To do oxygen treatments successfully, it must be continued in sequence and frequency to get deeper and deeper into tissues and into the brain. It is difficult in some areas of the country to find a doctor or clinic that has hyperbaric tanks for health related uses versus the gigantic ones they have at hospitals that are cost prohibitive.

To take oxygen farther into the brain, you can even breathe pure oxygen while on a treadmill or while exercising. The increase in heart rate and blood flow while breathing pure oxygen will push it deeper into the tissues to promote healing.

Scuba diving itself is an even better form of this because you are actually physically changing the pressure and oxygen flow, rather than having it simulated in a chamber.

Section 5- Essential Oils

At the Lyme treatment facility they use Young Living essential oils. Young Living sells the purest forms of essential oils on the market. They are so pure they can be ingested internally as well. I experienced them for the first time there where they diffuse them often right in the lobby and the doctors use them topically in treatment.

These oils are powerful and unbelievable. Their uses seem almost endless for an unfathomable list of ailments. The pocket guide is a wonderful tool for navigating how to develop a protocol. From sleep, to brain regeneration to heart attitude, to healing and complete reversal of symptoms – these oils are up to the task.

I would have been using these all along if I had known about them. For behavior, emotional balancing, energy, sleep, allergies, cleaning, and overall healing. I am still incorporating different usages of these into our lives and am still discovering more and more ways they are successful.

I use Peace and Calming for stress and emotional upsets. We diffuse Thieves oil often for killing of bacteria/viruses/pathogens in the air or our bodies. In fact, this is the one I use to clean the house with, counters/sinks/showers/toilets and floors. Frankincense and

Lavender are excellent for promoting healing and overall wellness. There are specific targeted oil groups for brain function, hormones, cell memory, etc.

I have recently begun using Brain Power to help restore my brain function after so much ammonia and blood flow problems. I also use Cedarwood and Citrus Fresh at times for increased brain function and processing. It is amazing how much better my A to B strings of thought have become mentally using these oils. I also use a couple of drops of lemon oil in my water at breakfast and it gives me the boost of energy I used to get with caffeine.

When the kids are fighting, I diffuse Mister oil, Peace and Calming, or Transformation for immediate changes in attitude and behavior.

From a spiritual and emotional perspective, I apply Release oil when I am feeling resentment or harboring anger or frustration from this disease and the toil it has taken on our family.

Whatever symptoms you are feeling or experiencing, these oils can help you. See the resources section.

Section 6- Environmental Testing

Examine random testing for radon, mold, other toxins, etc. in your home, school or work environment. We accidently found mold after 11 months of treatment, we were doing great and went to stay with a family member. After being at their house for 10 minutes, my daughter started coughing and turned into a psychotic mess. After two days and two nights, it got worse and worse. We did detox baths and finally I resorted to the asthma medicine which helped a little. Why would the asthma medicine help was the real question? We loaded all up in the car for the 8 hours home and she turned into a little angel and quit coughing.

They got mold testing done at their house and found a bunch, the black bad stuff. On a hunch and acting on paranoia, I had our house tested and found some in the laundry room and guest room from old water leaks and covering the insulation of the AC coil blowing mold spores into the entire house every time we kicked the AC or heat on in the house. Take notice on whether or not the symptoms increase or decrease when outside, or at school or at someone's house. It was not that expensive to call and get mold inspection. Put your suspicions to rest and pay to have the tests done.

You cannot reach complete healing if the immune system is still being stressed in your environment – that includes the school. I also know children that are so sensitive to smells and light that the type of bulbs used in the classroom affect their concentration. One parent I know got their school to have a "no smell" zone. NO teacher or parent or worker could wear smelly perfumes or lotions while in the school building. We do this now for peanuts, why not for chemical toxic smells. Some schools use 6000k full spectrum florescent lights which improves child behavior and learning.

Let your mind wander to all the places and ways that toxins could be affecting your condition. Did your office just install new carpet? Is the building where you work considered a "sick" building? How could you find this out? I would pay for the air tests myself if where I work or where my children go to school is exacerbating the problem.

Electro Magnetic Fields (EMFs) are becoming an increasing problem for the chronic sick population. One of my lyme friends has seizures when she enters places with giant Wifi. Consider turning off your wifi at home at night, and don't sleep with your phone or other electronics on your nightstand.

You will not heal no matter what the treatment if you are in a toxic environment.

In your everyday environment, think twice before letting the carwash place put a fragrance into your car after they wash and vacuum it. Hang up your dry cleaning in the garage or outside and let it off gas the chemicals before bringing them into the house. Ask the lady in the cubicle next to you at work to take a short vacation from the perfume or candle scents she has going full blast. Or ask to be moved. Talk to the schools where your kids go about going "scent free".

If you are into candles, buy the natural bees wax candles. Stop using your Scentsy. Unplug the Glade Plug-ins. Take that smelly pink thing out of the toilet. Don't spray Febreeze on anything. Quit putting fabric sheets in your dryer and using perfume. All your old habits are about to change, take notice of them all and make adjustments where necessary.

Section 7- CCSVI - Chronic Cerebrospinal Venous Insufficiency

CCSVI - Chronic Cerebrospinal Venous Insufficiency is a condition that in the last four years has been discovered to be associated with Multiple Schelorisis (MS) by Dr. Paulo Zamboni in 2008 after 10 years of research. It is so new; they are not sure what causes it and how to prevent it. The supposition in regard to Lyme is that the bacteria or a co-infection causes some sort of sticky material that cinches down the venous flow out of the brain.

In the United States, the first case of CCSVI treatment protocols were pioneered by Dr. Michael Dake of Stanford University. Dr. E. Mark Haacke of Wayne State University, McMaster University, the Brain Body Institute, and the MRI Institute for Biomedical Research, is at the forefront of developing CCSVI imaging protocols, and, particularly iron quantification. Dr. Robert Zivadinov of the Buffalo Neuroimaging Analysis Center at the University of Buffalo is leading clinical trials testing the relationship between CCSVI and MS, and the efficacy of CCSVI treatment (from CCSVI Alliance).

These architects on the cutting edge of medical breakthroughs have designed the MRI software and ultrasound components to find and diagnose CCSVI. So why couldn't I just walk into any MRI facility and ask them to look for CCSVI? Well, first of all they would have to know what it is and how to look for it. Even if they were familiar with CCSVI, their MRI machines are not "programmed" to find it.

Depending on where you are in the country, it will be difficult to locate a doctor who has even heard of this issue. Finding someone who can then actually find it is another challenge entirely. So many people asked why I not only had to go all the way to Las Vegas to correct it, but to also an MRI facility to find it. Because I had to find a place that spoke the "language" and understood what they were even looking for in the first place. Research the places performing this intervention and protocol and call and ask questions. The MRI software used to find CCSVI is only used in a few facilities in the country.

The treatment center I went to in Las Vegas was designed and programmed by Dr. Haacke. They work in conjunction with an outpatient surgical facility where the CCSVI surgeon who got her experience on MS patients in Buffalo, NY.

There are only a few surgeons in the entire country (Newport Beach, CA, Las Vegas, NV and Atlanta, GA) actually correcting CCSVI and in the last 2 years or so, they realized there was a crossover from MS to Lyme and other neurological conditions. The surgeon in Las Vegas who performed my surgery has performed the surgery on thousands of MS patients, but only a scant handful of Lymies. It is that new. But, it was that successful.

Now enter Lyme into the CCSVI conundrum with the introduction of Dr. Dietrich Klighardt. Dr. Klinghardt MD, PhD, is Founder of the Klinghardt Academy (USA), the American Academy of Neural Therapy, Medical Director of the Institute of Neurobiology, and lead clinician at the Sophia Health Institute, located in Woodinville, Washington. He is also Founder and Chairman of the Institute for Neurobiology (Germany) and (Switzerland). Klinghardt Academy (USA) provides teachings to the English speaking world on biological interventions and Autonomic Response Testing assessment techniques.

In "A Deep Look Beyond Lyme" from 2011 in Redmond, WA. - Dr. Klinghardt spoke on CCSVI and LYME.

- Dr. Klinghardt has seen CCSVI in 100% of his tested MS patients, autism patients, Parkinson's patients, ALS patients, and Lyme patients.
- There are 5 parameters that are looked at during a CCSVI evaluation. In MS, 2 of 5 are often observed. In Lyme, it has been closer to 4 of 5 and in autism, it is often 5 of 5. The best Lyme patient thus far was 3 of 5. Lyme patients, on average, test worse than MS patients.

I was improving but continually backsliding and the heart palpitations and chest pain was getting incredibly intense the better I felt. It wasn't until after I had this surgery performed that my true recovery began, because the Lyme treatment was not reaching my brain due to the insufficient blood flow.

Take this very seriously and find a doctor who understands it. I don't know the actual percentages, but nearly half of the Lymies I've met have CCSVI.

Specifically, Dr. Zamboni hypothesized that CCSVI could damage CNS tissue in a variety of ways, notably by breaching the blood brain barrier of stressed, dilated, and inflamed blood vessels, and leaking iron and other antigens into nearby tissues. His team began treating MS patients with a technique known as Percutaneous Balloon Angioplasty (PTA).

Today, based on Dr. Zamboni's findings and his theory of CCSVI, doctors in the United States, Europe, South Asia, and the Middle East have begun treating venous obstructions by using either PTA, stents, or both. Further, independent research is currently underway attempting to confirm, or refute, the link between CCSVI and MS as well as the efficacy of CCSVI treatment.(from CCSVI Alliance)

Section 8 - Bach Flower

The doctor who developed these flower remedies comes from the general idea as the Young Living brand. God put healing properties in all his creation for us to discover. Dr. Bach discovered these 38 flowers had healing emotional properties relative to stress, environment, trauma and sleep. The company produces a few varied remedies that are called "Rescue Remedy", "Sleep Remedy" and "Rescue Energy". They come in various forms from tincture to cream, spray and gum.

The general Rescue Remedy works great. I carry one in my purse and have one on every floor of the house. In fact, it is usually my first go to. If it can't clear it out, then it's a deeper toxic issue or pathogen. In the emotional instability of Lyme, I highly recommend having this remedy nearby for a go to whenever the tears begin and won't end. Also, depression can hit Lyme patients hard core. If that is you, go online to bachflower.com and in the individual list for what each flower essense helps, read them and find the one that speaks to you and order it and give it freely to yourself.

We had our chiropractor/kinesiologist using energetic testing, pinpoint the exact flower that is the most beneficial for each member of our family and we use that specific remedy just for them. If you don't have access to this, on the Bach flower website (see resource list), they list summaries for each flower remedy and what they typically help. It might give you some guidance on which to purchase if you want something with more punch for your loved one.

Check out the Bach Flower website. It lists all the flower remedies, the symptoms present and their curative purposes.

For instance, I am administering Impatiens to myself often lately. I believe it is helping to tame the "Lyme rage" I have been experiencing. It also reads like a go to remedy for anyone like me who has high expectations and a low tolerance for chaos that follows both my kids and their school activities around.

Section 9- Co-Infections

I can only scratch the surface and don't have a great and well-rounded understanding of co-infections except that I had a slew of them. I haven't met a Lymie yet who didn't. But they are all varied and inconsistent in how they impact each body with the Lyme itself. What is certain, however, is that the Lyme spirochete bacteria are good at getting the party started. It creates an environment and a toxic hierarchy in which all other pathogens thrive.

Co-infections – Other pathogens that can be carried with the Lyme spirochete into the body simultaneously that can also cause damage and fatalities. Babesia, Bartonella, Ehrlichia, Colorado Tick Fever, Tick Relapsing Fever, Q Fever, Flavivirus, Rocky Mountain Spotted Fever, West Nile Virus, Tularemia, Micoplasma

Again, make sure the doctors you see fully understand co-infections and don't glaze over when you mention mycoplasma. It is like an onion, each step of healing peels another layer of toxins and pathogens out of your system. Sometimes new symptoms can erupt and all of a sudden you have a parasite or virus going crazy that was not "there" before or evident in any test. It was dormant or possibly suppressed by the other pathogens or your own immune system.

I highly suggest doing some additional reading and listening on YouTube.com to Dr. Klinghardt on the Klinghardt Academy website - http://www.klinghardtacademy.com. Dr. Mercola's website is also a good resource for additional information, at least to start with. I'm also incredibly proud of some fellow Lymies who created http://slyme.tiredoflyme.com/index.html which is a search engine powered by Google, but only searches out previously registered Lyme websites for the information.

Of course, I'm biased and believe that Dr. David Jernigan's book on Lyme Disease – Beating Lyme Disease is a must read and packed with technical and scientific information about Lyme and the body that I can't begin to know and understand.

Section 10- Diet Restrictions

Okay don't freak out here – this could get extensive and overwhelming. Don't let it make you drown. Eating good is what can save you here. It's time to take a serious look at what you are inputting into your body. It's the fuel in which your body can fight off infection and heal. Are you putting in premium food or only sometimes? I looked at it this way; I would rather live thousands of more days with energy and vigor and really live than eat gluten or ding dongs or ice cream whenever I want.

Yes, I have to really hunt for restaurants I can eat out in, but there are more choices now than there ever used to be. I miss some of my favorite foods, but I would rather live than dwell on it. And I do allow myself some guilty pleasures from time to time. They are just more infrequent and toned down from before.

First things first – your body needs all the energy it can, so do not put any drugs or alcohol into your system. Your liver is already doing a mighty deed to try to filter out all the other toxins produced from all the pathogens in your body, it does not need to also filter out the 4 glasses of wine on the weekend. Also take care on the ingestion of over-the-counter medication unless absolutely necessary. That includes, Motrin, Advil, Claritin, etc. Try to find an alternative natural or homeopathic solution to save your body.

Secondly, take a serious look at the Feingold diet as a starting place. It is not quite as intimidating as going gluten free, dairy free or Paleo diets. Go to Feingold.org and check out the major things to avoid.

Dr. Feingold wrote a book called "Why is Your Child Hyperactive" detailing the history of these food dyes. It is fascinating – let me give you a synopsis. They were originally made as fabric dyes out of coal tar in the late 18th century. There were dozens of them. They flooded the food market with them at the turn of the century and it caused such rampant disease and death that they removed them all but 9. We are the only country left in the Westernized world that still allows them in food. They have been banned in EU, Japan, Canada, etc. So when you Kraft makes their Mac-N-Cheese for export, they omit the dye and use something plant based, but not so in the good ole US of A. We say "we love that yellow dye" bring it on.

The most important is to avoid these dyes, preservatives, MSG, high fructose corn syrup, nitrates and artificial flavors. This doesn't mean you have to miss out on your favorites foods, it just means you will be shopping in a different area of the store for them or ordering them online if you have no local resource. For instance, the granola you buy, you can find an organic substitute that doesn't use HFCS or preservatives. The crackers or ice cream bars, same thing. If you cannot find them in the organic section of your grocery store, then go to a health food store and pay a bit more for a while or eat them less often. Super Target and Super WalMart in my home town have a surprising amount of organic options. Do your research.

If you cannot find a local source, then make a monthly road trip to a city with a Whole Foods Market or Trader Joes. I also use the Amazon super saver to order stuff online and get free shipping in bulk amounts. The hardest thing to remember is to avoid those processed meats with nitrates. Boar's Head lunch meats are gluten free and most of them are free of nitrates. They even have a completely "uncured" ham option that my kids love. Both my grocery store and Target carry brand of bacon that is uncured.

If you don't have a grocery store carrying it, request it. You never know. A health food store will also likely carry Applegate Farms or other brands of uncured hotdogs, pepperoni, summer sausage, and other lunch meats. There are oodles of options.

As for the dye thing, all organic foods are using natural food dyes out of plants/vegetables. Last time I read the labels, Goldfish crackers (regular) were the only crackers in the normal cracker aisle that didn't use synthetic dye to make them orange.

The preservatives and artificial flavors are using the same type of petroleum base that the dyes are so our bodies cannot process that petroleum. It ends up in brain tissue causes all kinds of neurological harm. You want to conspiracy theory, think about the surge of Alzheimer's and Autism in the past 100 years since we've been using these in food and "modernizing" our diets.

Okay, off my soapbox now. Use the Feingold website for the list of all the "trick" names of the preservatives. Using the dye free Motrin is better than with dye for instance, but the benzoate preservative and artificial flavors still make my kids crazy. In fact, my son was so sensitive to benzoate at one time that we couldn't find a sunscreen in the world that he wouldn't react to. So we have not literally used a stitch of sunscreen in over 4 years, with not one sunburn. Another cultural taboo debunked.

Go organic. I know it sounds expensive. Each step of this requires more money. Do it a little bit at a time. Use the following guide for the Dirty Dozen and the Clean 15 to tell you what to buy organic and what to buy conventional. Go to your local farmer's market and get better deals. Grown your own garden and can stuff for the winter. Do a farm share. There are many options for savings, including Azure Standard and Bountiful Baskets.

Dirty Dozen - Apples, Celery, Sweet bell peppers, Peaches, Strawberries, Nectarines, Grapes, Spinach, Lettuce, Cucumbers, Blueberries, and Potatoes

Clean Fifteen - Onion, Sweet corn, Pineapples, Avocado, Cabbage, Sweet peas, Asparagus, Mangoes, Eggplant, Kiwi, Cantaloupe, Sweet potatoes, Grapefruit, Watermelon, and Mushrooms

Your body does not need the extra chemicals to process with each conventional apple you ingest. If you do buy conventional, consider soaking/washing with a mixture of grapefruit seed extract and water to kill off pathogens and wash off chemicals and wax.

Meat. Check your sources for meat. Look for a local butcher in town and ask what's in the meat. He might look at you funny or he might surprise you by answering right away. Most butcher shops across the country have closed, but the remaining ones are setting themselves apart from the grocery store meat by supplying free range, antibiotic free chicken, grass fed beef, lamb and many other options.

If you are not going to make the shift to organic meat, then lessen your intake. Especially in red meats. Go grass fed or go home. Google for private farms near you that you can buy meat in bulk direct. Your local farmer's market is a great resource for this in pork, chicken, deer, buffalo, and grass fed beef.

Try juicing or making shakes. It's amazing what organic veggies juiced can do for your body. Especially if you are in a low spot or having a particularly hard day. Go directly to juicing with almond or rice milk with your veggies and fruit. What you put in is what you get out. A friend of mine helped her husband through a terrible leg pain illness by juicing carrots and celery every day. They went through 20 lbs. of carrots and 5 lbs. of celery each week.

Now brace yourself. This is the hardest for most people. Nothing gets people more fired up in our culture than trying to take away their sugar and bread. Let's talk sugar. We'll get the sweets out of the way first. No, you do not have to give up anything sweet for the rest of your life. It is true that your body will heal faster without the agitation of sugar to the Candida in your gut, but some sweeteners aren't as toxic to your body. We use organic brown rice syrup as a substitute for corn syrup in recipes. From time to time now, we use organic cane sugar when we need powdered sugar or brown sugar for a recipe. The kids have to have icing on their birthday cakes once a year or what kind of mom would I be? Date sugar or dates and coconut can be used in recipes as a natural sweetener and apple juice concentrate is even used in some of my recipe books to feed your sweet tooth in a muffin or cake. No, they don't all taste the same and don't all behave in your recipes similarly, but they do taste good and you will get used to something sweet that isn't made from processed to the hilt crappy white cane sugar.

Since I am hitting below the knees we are going for bread and cheese next. Gluten, casein and soy molecules are all very negative to the immune system and autoimmune disease with Leaky Gut Syndrome. The body can be confused by these food molecules and attack different body tissue as invaders. With an overactive and weakened immune system, since we eat one or all of these at each meal. It is imperative to go GFCFSF (Gluten Free Casein Free Soy Free) to help the immune system actually fight the real bad guys. We have gotten to such a place in our culture that we "do" more things to the food than has ever been done before in history. Did you know that if you fed milk from the grocery store to a calf it would kill it?

Goat's milk, by the molecule, is the closest to human breast milk and is the safest for us to ingest. We have access to quality goat's cheese, yogurt, cream cheese and milk. Ease into the goat and sheep cheese arena to substitute instead of cow's milk. Or if you are really lucky and don't live in CA where they are trying to make it illegal, find a local small dairy that you can buy raw milk and raw milk products from. The human body can process them in the raw form much easier, and by the way, it is delicious.

Almond milk is probably the best substitute. Rice milk is a bit less expensive than Almond Milk. Both are good to cook with and drink. Ease into the pool on this. Don't freak yourself out by trying to love a nice tall glass of Rice Milk with your organic cookie and think your taste buds won't say "weird" right off the bat. But do it gradually, like putting it over your cereal, cooking muffins with it. Use it for a creamer in your coffee, etc. These are great ways of getting used to it gradually. Your kids might like the vanilla or chocolate versions of both of these milks. They do have more sugar than the regular versions, so we don't do them anymore, or use them sparingly. I certainly wouldn't cook with the sugary versions as they might disrupt your recipe.

I went there and raided your bread closet and took it all out. It's terrible and will be the most disruptive thing I could ever do to your diet. You will be amazed at how you feel though. I strongly suggest you do a detox or cleanse diet on your way into going GF. It will help cleanse your gut and palette from gluten. There are no perfect substitutes for gluten. That being said, you can find or create a good flour blend with the right amounts of binders included (xanthum gum, guar gum, agar powder). These binders along with the proper amount of starch flour (arrowroot, tapioca, mandioca, potato) will give some elasticity to the bread or product you are making. Look for the gluten free bread products in the freezer, Udi's is our favorite. The bread mixes on the shelves are all pretty good also, including the brownie mixes, cakes, pancakes, etc.

For pancakes, sweet breads and cakes, you can do an almost direct swap out of regular flour and gluten free flour. If you do this, you might need to add some extra or lessen the amount of liquid depending on what flours you use. An extra egg might be necessary for more binding in cookies or dough, but most sweet breads are fine with the recipe designated amount (see "Eating Your Way Through Lyme" cookbook for more details.)

Now, on a non-food note, don't forget to look for the dyes and preservatives outside your pantry. I found out that the clear hand soap refill I bought from the store had blue and red dye in it – to make it clear? My laundry detergent, toothpaste, shampoo, lotion – all had dye in it. If you are going to ingest it, smell it or wear it, read the label. Deodorants and antiperspirants use aluminum which is not a great thing to be ingesting in your state either. You can find natural substitutes out there for those too.

It seems daunting, but I make my own laundry soap and dishwasher soap or honestly you could use baking soda and Thieves oil and that would work fine. One of my girlfriends uses vinegar.

There are many products online and in health food stores for shampoos, deodorants, toothpastes and products without dyes, preservatives or artificial flavors. You don't have to throw out the whole lot at once unless you are really sick or one of your kids is. Just replace as you empty what you have.

For example, when I started this undertaking, I took a trusty sharpie marker and put a giant X on the back and front of any product that the kids were not to eat or use. That way my husband and all who entered the house (grandparents, babysitters) would know not to give those to the kids. We ate up and used up all the "bad" stuff and gave the kids the new stuff right away.

Section 11- Exercise, Positive Thinking and Support

Physical exercise is an imperative part of the journey to healing. What is it you enjoy doing, walking, running, canoeing, and swimming? Start slow and find a "partner" to exercise with you. It is motivating to have someone who is pushing you to keep trying even when it is hard or difficult. Also, someone to keep you from pushing too hard. I felt better having someone to "spot" me on the days that were somewhat questionable if I should be operating heavy machinery and getting out in the world with an increased heart rate.

It's also a wonderful opportunity for fellowship. My first acts of exercise began with prayer walking with my mentor at church twice a week. The ability to incorporate positive thinking with exercise has been invaluable to my healing.

There are books on CD or online radio options for inputting positive reinforcement and uplifting material into the mind during the healing process. It is a battle to keep the mind focused on a spirit of thankfulness in the pit of despair. So even when you cannot, input uplifting music and positive talk to help reprogram your mind.

Countless studies have proven that the thoughts of the mind help determine the actions of the physical self in a state of chronic illness. Your negative thoughts and emotions can largely determine your rate of ascent out of this pit. Build up your emotional self with your physical self.

Neurofeedback is a cutting edge technology that helps "reprogram" thinking and attitude. Some other patients I have met through Hansa have used this technique. Neurofeedback is a type of biofeedback that uses electroencephalography (EEG) to provide a signal that can be used by a person to receive feedback about brain activity. The EEG signal is fed into computer software first then the feedback, usually a movie or music, is returned to the person being trained. This feedback loop can produce changes in brainwave activity. The process used to adjust brainwave activity is known as operant conditioning, which is a method where rewards for positive behavior increase learning capabilities.

The concept is fairly simple. The computer monitors your brainwaves while you watch a movie or listen to music. When deviations from normal brainwave activity occur, the computer triggers an audio or visual cue that alerts the patient that they are outside normal ranges.

Training the brain using neurofeedback can change these brainwaves over time, adjusting them into normal, healthy ranges. It can improve alertness, attention, emotional regulation, behavior, cognitive function, and mental flexibility. When the brain moves back into normal ranges, users will often see a reduction in symptoms. The best part of neurofeedback is that results are often permanent, allowing a person to reduce or even eliminate medications altogether.

Another methodology available that I have not personally experienced, but I know people who have gotten positive results from is The EVOX. The EVOX facilitates a process called Perception Reframing. Perception is the way you feel and think about something. Because we perceive more than we are aware of, perception is more often 'felt' rather than 'thought about.'

EVOX uses the voice (VOX is Latin for voice) to map perception about specific topics like health, relationships, work or athletic performance; any aspect of life. It then analyses that map, called a Perception Index, and creates a playback information packet that the body uses to bring perception to the level of awareness and allow it to be reframed. EVOX is used to improve every aspect of human performance.

In the case of relationships, a person may repeatedly attract destructive behaviors; for example, the woman who repeatedly marries abusive men. Even though at an intellectual level she knows better, for some reason she continues to fall for 'the wrong guy.' This is the result of a static perception that perpetuates dysfunctional outcomes and has very little to do with her intellectual desire for something better.

Counseling is also a great platform to explore during chronic Lyme for you and your spouse or kids. Chronic illness is rough on the entire family, so having someone unpack that for you can be immeasurable. My counselor did amazing work helping me unravel the death's door fear and struggle I had. It seems weird to talk to a stranger about it, but it might very well be the proper way to completely be open about how you feel or have felt. It the chronic illness has taken its toll on relationships, take them into the session with you and find out how others perceive you in the illness. Seeing yourself from their point of view can alter how you approach each day mentally, spiritually and emotionally.

Support. I know it is humbling and difficult to ask, but you must ask. This Lyme thing is a beast to fight off and the battle is long and hard. People need to know how bad it is and they need to be able to help. Make a list of the things you can't get accomplished and give them to your neighbor/friend/family member or church so they can help. For me, it was driving, cooking, grocery shopping, helping with the kids and cleaning house. I had an army of women helping hold my household together. And if I had actually asked more often, the army would have been even bigger.

One last thing that seems like an age old concept, but works brilliantly. Get a mentor or accountability partner. Maybe its someone who has battled Lyme disease and is farther up the healing ladder than you are, maybe it is an heart friend, or a neighbor, coworker or spiritual friend. You need someone who can keep you looking forward and upward and fighting ahead. Someone who will compassionately listen, hug you, love on you, but give you truth when you need to hear it.

Section 12- Anointing and Prayer

I cannot begin to stress enough how positive thinking and prayer can help through this battle of Lyme. For more information on prayer through healing, please read My God, My Lyme. It is a detailed story of my spiritual journey through Lyme and healing. I list many scriptures and resource books to help with positive thinking and how to walk through the "valley of the shadow of death" and make it to the other side a better person.

What I want to touch on here is the biblical anointing for healing. Hyssop oil is mentioned several times in the Old and New Testaments for use in prayer for healing, consecration, protection and worship. Frankincense oil also has many healing properties and was used throughout the bible. Do your own research and look into the Twelve Oils of Ancient Scripture that Young Living sells.

Research the biblical applications for anointing and healing and the laying of hands.

> *So Samuel took the horn of oil and anointed him in the presence of his brothers, and from that day on the Spirit of the Lord came powerfully upon David. (1 Samuel 16:13)*
>
> *Now this I know: The Lord gives victory to his anointed. He answers him from his heavenly sanctuary with the victorious power of his right hand. (Psalm 20:6)*
>
> *I have found David my servant; with my sacred oil I have anointed him. (Psalm 89:20)*

They drove out many demons and anointed many sick people with oil and healed them. (Mark 6:13)

You prepare a table before me in the presence of my enemies. You anoint my head with oil; my cup overflows. (Psalm 23:5)

Always be clothed in white, and always anoint your head with oil. (Ecclesiastes 9:8)

Is anyone among you sick? Let them call the elders of the church to pray over them and anoint them with oil in the name of the Lord. (James 5:14)

And the people all tried to touch him, because power was coming from him and healing them all. (Luke 6:19)

Then a man who is ceremonially clean is to take some hyssop, dip it in the water and sprinkle the tent and all the furnishings and the people who were there. (Numbers 19:18)

Cleanse me with hyssop, and I will be clean; wash me, and I will be whiter than snow. (Psalm 51:7)

Then Moses took the anointing oil and anointed the tabernacle and everything in it, and so consecrated them. (Leviticus 8:10)

You love righteousness and hate wickedness; therefore God, your God, has set you above your companions by anointing you with the oil of joy. (Psalm 45:7)

In my book My God, My Lyme, chapter 21 is completely centered around claiming the scriptural promises of God. There is such power in praying scripture and using it to help elevate our mind and emotions when we feel we are too weak to do it alone.

Section 13 - Journal It

Keep a journal or record of symptoms and release and any new ones along the way. You will become such an expert of every nook and cranny of the body, almost to a fault. Each of these slight and major shifts indicates something different to a doctor. Document them and keep track. It is also helpful to look back and be encouraged by improvement.

Your advocate or family member or spouse will find it helpful to fully understand how you feel. They can also use your list of questions to ask on your behalf when they go with you to the doctor. There is nothing more frustrating than getting home from expensive doctor appointment that you waited weeks to get to and forget to ask 2 of the questions you had for him/her.

No matter how many times we try to tell those loved ones around us what is actually going on and how we feel, written words penetrate much deeper. And for the times and days we shield them from how bad it is, someday they should know and can read it.

On the path to healing there will be setbacks. It is inevitable – not a matter of if but when. They will happen. One step forward and two steps back some days. It is imperative that you have a journal to go back and remember how far you have come and how bad you used to feel. Our pain receptors have a strange memory for how terrific our tolerance of the illness.

I wholeheartedly believe that it is therapeutic to write it down and get the emotions that come with it out. Whether you are facebooking the journey, blogging it, handwriting it or typing it – or a combination of all of those. Just do it. You will truly feel improved to get it out.

Section 14- Autonomic Nervous System

The Autonomic Nervous System is the part of the peripheral nervous system that acts as a control system, functioning largely below the level of consciousness, and controls visceral functions. The ANS affects heart rate, digestion, respiratory rate, salivation, perspiration, pupillary dilation, micturition (urination), and sexual arousal. Bottom line is that the ANS controls fight or flight or your body's reaction to anything dangerous or painful. Most autonomous functions are involuntary but a number of ANS actions can work alongside some degree of conscious control. Everyday examples include breathing, swallowing, and sexual arousal, and in some cases functions such as heart rate.

The Lyme bacteria release deadly neurotoxins and ammonia during its life cycle. Neurotoxins are an extensive class of exogenous chemical neurological insults which can adversely affect function in both developing and mature nervous tissue.

The ammonia and neurotoxins plague the ANS within the chronic Lymie wreaking havoc in various symptoms. The poisoning toxicity has tremendous damage throughout many systems and organs in the body like a domino effect from the ANS all the way down. All things that affect

Lymies in various forms of pain and struggle with could be caused by neurotoxins and ammonia poisoning to the ANS.

There are various forms of cutting edge therapies that can help reroute, reset and "reboot" the ANS after treating and healing from the Lyme. It is imperative that the rebooting of the ANS happen in proper sequence in the healing so the body can learn to communicate properly again.

Life Vessels and Synchronicity are the two therapies I have experienced. The Life Vessel therapy uses light, sound, color and vibration in combination to relax and reboot the ANS. My entire family has experienced success with the Life Vessels. (see resource page)

Section 15- Adrenals

The Adrenal glands are part of the endocrine system that sit at the top of the kidneys and are mainly responsible for releasing hormones in response to stress through the making cortisol, and adrenaline.

Adrenal insufficiency occurs when the adrenal glands are subjected to intense prolonged stress, I.E. during a chronic illness.

If not treated, adrenal insufficiency may result in severe abdominal pains, vomiting, profound muscle weakness and fatigue, depression, extremely low blood pressure, weight loss, kidney failure, changes in mood and personality, and shock. An adrenal crisis often occurs if the body is subjected to stress, such as an accident, injury, surgery, chronic illness or severe infection.

In my case, my adrenal insufficiency was also brought on by my pituitary gland malfunctioning and not producing correct hormones. In theory, due to my symptoms from onset to healing, my pituitary housed a great deal of ammonia from Lyme.

Adrenal insufficiency can also occur, like in my case, when the hypothalamus or the pituitary gland does not make adequate amounts of the hormones that aid in regulating adrenal function. This is called secondary adrenal insufficiency and is caused by lack of production of

ACTH in the pituitary or lack of CRH in the hypothalamus. From top to bottom, my adrenals were not getting stimulated correctly and were burnt out from prolonged stressors.

Adrenal Fatigue is another commonly used terminology that is widely undiagnosed and pervasive throughout Lyme. Most commonly associated with intense or prolonged stress, it can also arise in chronic infections. The fatigue in adrenal fatigue is not relieved by sleep and is very hard to pinpoint and find causes. People experiencing adrenal fatigue often have to use coffee, colas, and other stimulants to get going in the morning and prop themselves up during the day.

In my case, I wasn't having to prop up as much as I couldn't get my adrenals to wind down. It was like they were stuck on panic - red lined, especially at night. My heart would race and skip and dance and pound for hours leaving me unable to sleep or even rest. Which would leave me exhausted for the next day in which all I could do was lay around and sleep.

In extreme cases, like mine, you may have difficulty getting out of bed for more than a few hours in each day. With each increment of reduction in adrenal function, every organ and system in your body is more profoundly affected. Changes occur in your metabolism, fluid and electrolyte balance, heart and cardiovascular system and even sex drive. Many other alterations take place at the biochemical and cellular levels in response to and to compensate for the decrease in adrenal hormones that occurs with adrenal fatigue. Your body does its best to make up for and borrow when the adrenals fail to act, but it does so at a price.

As you can see, if you add this layer in on top of the already struggling Lyme disease, the symptoms are going to be erratic and all over the board. The organs are going to begin to fail one by one in chronic inflammation. Herein lies the extreme dangers for Lymies.

Talk to your doctor about Adrenal problems. A well-trained Naturopath, Chiropractor or Lyme Physician will know how to test for low adrenal function and help prop them up with supplements, and get you functioning better and on the road to healing.

Section 16- Post Lyme Syndrome and Prevention

Post Lyme Syndrome (PLS) is not a phrase you will hear many doctors talk about and certainly you can't even find much under a Google search, but ask any Lymie and you know that it exists.

I have heard described to me what happens to an amputee patient after the trauma. They still have pain in the missing appendage. Phantom pain. How is it that the brain and nerves register pain in something that is not there anymore? Memory. Your brain is not the only place that stores memories. Each cell in your body stores memories. Cell memory.

In Post Lyme Syndrome has many facets, and one is this cell memory. For months (and even still today) after I had no ammonia in my body, no trace of the active spirochete called Lyme, I would have the same symptoms at various times. After painting the kitchen cabinets, after walking three days in a row, before my menstrual cycle would begin.

Why on earth would my body register Lyme symptoms instead of tired muscles? Lyme symptoms instead of menstrual cramps? Cell memory.

When the body has been in a chronic health state, all the last settings were on "panic" or "all hands on deck". So, initially when the body needs to react to something, it calls up its last setting and registers it instead. So, if any severe emotional, spiritual or physical occurrence, the body can misfire the symptoms.

So, I realize you have already been through too much with the realization of having Lyme and fighting Lyme. Now you have to endure the Post Lyme Syndrome too? Well, for each of us it is different. It does usually register in the most critical organ – most likely ground zero for the Lyme.

Any stress on the body, whether physical, psychological or toxic, will activate the sympathetic nervous system, a function of the Autonomic Nervous System (ANS), and create what is referred to as "a fight or flight response". This could be the result of a car accident, surgery, emotional distress, fear, toxic exposure or any threat or perceived threat to life or of injury. In a natural healing response, once the stress is removed, the nervous system should reset itself. Unfortunately, for many people the modern stresses are so great and continuous, there may be no chance for the body to return itself to normal. A local area then becomes locked into a constant fight or flight or "freeze" state. This area becomes a disturbance field and can for many years interfere with the normal nervous system regulation in the body

Talk to your doctor about this and methods for "rebooting" the Autonomic Nervous System. A good "reboot" will help clear out the body's memory for the "red-lined" panic it wants to feel. The ANS is the "control" panel for all the functions conscious and unconscious of the nervous system. If during the chronic stages of the Lyme, the signals got crossed or have misfired, a "reboot" will help the systems get the right signals. Overstimulation from sounds, lights, temperature – all are very familiar to the Lymie. Bright colors even "hurt" my eyes and made my brain malfunction. It was critical to my ability to read again to have the rebooting and retraining.

Once, after a series of retraining exercises for my ANS with the doctor I was doing almost a physical sobriety test standing by the table in his office to check my cross brain function. He asked me to begin to march. I did and it felt funny and after he stifled laughter (and later I did too), he explained it felt weird because I was marching left hand with left foot and right hand with right foot. My brain was so dysfunctional, it was registering marching backwards. I knew it felt weird too, but couldn't pinpoint why. That is just a pale example of PLS (Post Lyme Syndrome) and the affects it has on the ANS and why it has to be reset and retrained.

Yes, it is very much like what physical therapy for a stroke victim is like depending on what symptoms you have. The physical/sound/light sensors can be retrained in therapy. But what about the organs? There are many different available forms of ANS support available and your doctor might know of some that I am not familiar with or have heard of. Check into acupuncture and neurophotonics (sound and light therapy) in your area and for your needs.

In addition, supporting the adrenals and checking in on the workings of the entire endocrine system, which is responsible for how your body responds to stress. Most likely, even without the Lyme targeting the adrenals, they are cashed out because of all the stress on the body emotionally and physically to be chronically ill. Most doctors can do saliva or blood tests to determine how to prop up the endocrine system and get it regulating more normally and supplementing until it recovers.

Section 17- Pregnancy and Lyme

Without question, I can tell you that despite medical testing and supplemental medical journals, Lyme disease can be passed in the womb to your baby. I know personally of a handful of mothers who unknowingly passed Lyme disease and its co-infections to all their kids, including myself. My kids, after testing, had EVERY critter I did. Symptoms can show up right away or slowly over time. One mother I know only had one out of three of her kids show signs and she has never gotten sick herself. Lyme is like a tornado; it picks and chooses at random which family member will undergo destruction.

Talk to you doctor about the safe treatments you can undergo while pregnant; homeopathics, natural supplements and therapies that will protect your baby and help you and the baby be Lyme free.

Look for symptoms like constipation, diarrhea, excessive crying (colic), fever, sleeplessness, etc and talk to your LLMD doctor immediately when you see anything unusual in your baby.

Postscript

My journey and my valley are not over. Our family's battles continue but we have a winning record. We are chipping away at what Lyme has done in our home.

I am driving, I am reading, and I am writing. Most importantly, I am living. I am living, my eyes focused forward and upward. Trying to see all things He brings each day in light of the character building God is doing in our family.

We are still eating GFCFSF, but all the other sensitivities for the kids are gone. We eat goat's cheese now which is a delicacy in our house and we treasure it. The kids sleep through the night much better, way over half the time. The behavior problems have been severely diminished. My daughter doesn't complain of tummy aches anymore or launch into prepubescent "tearcapades" either.

If fact, I can't remember the last time she complained about a tummy ache. Wow. We have come a long way and as I write this, it is a good reminder to be thankful and continue the fight.

I have gained 25 lbs. back but still have about 5 to go and can't seem to put it on no matter how much GF dessert I eat (what a problem huh?). But my pants are no longer duct taped up and I can fit into most of my clothes again. I've even graduated away from the "butt pillow" which I had to use for over a year because I was so thin that it hurt to sit at the kitchen table in our wood chairs without padding.

When we have "regressions" with my son, I claim and remember these things He has accomplished and hold fast to the journey to fight and finish it off.

When I look in the mirror now I see a ton of more gray hairs, but I see life. I see my soul reflecting back a life that was worth fighting for and worth keeping.

My goal for myself and my kids is to live life to the full knowing that each breath is a gift from God. For us to use our talents and experiences to help others find hope and healing. In small measure, I pray for continued strength and for cow's cheese to re-enter our house to be devoured in late night snacks.

My son's goal is to someday eat Papa John's pizza. Maybe someday we will. But until then, I just found out a new pizza place down the street is serving gluten free pizza...

I would encourage each of you to journal this process. Document somehow, via Facebook, blog or writing how you survived and thrived in the valley. Let it be a testimony to others of God's faithfulness and goodness. Use this period in your life to help make His name great. Help other's struggling with Lyme or other debilitating illnesses or physical ailments. Tell Him to let Him use you to help others and to be that testimony. I call it being a Lyme evangelist. This Lyme disease is the most undiagnosed illness in our country. Help others identify and get on the right path. Pray for them. Encourage them.

Dear Friends, I pray that you may enjoy good health and that all may go well with you, even as your soul is getting along well. (3 John 2) I pray that the Lord will heal all your diseases (Psalm 103:3) and be your strength every morning and be your salvation in your distress. (Isaiah 33:2) I pray that for you who fear His name, the Sun of Righteousness will rise with healing in his wings. And you will go free, leaping with joy like calves let out to pasture. (Malachi 4:2) I pray that your suffering now is nothing compared to the glory God will reveal to you later. (Romans 8:18)

Glossary

Ammonia - is a compound of nitrogen and hydrogen with the formula NH3 . ammonia is both caustic and hazardous. It is a by product of the die off of Lyme disease and its co-infections.

Ammonia Toxicity - has been shown to induce swelling of astrocytes in the brain

Asperger's - is an autism spectrum disorder (ASD) that is characterized by significant difficulties in social interaction and nonverbal communication, alongside restricted and repetitive patterns of behavior and interests. It differs from other autism spectrum disorders by its relative preservation of linguistic and cognitive development. Although not required for diagnosis, physical clumsiness and atypical (peculiar, odd) use of language are frequently reported.

Autism Spectrum Disorder (ASD)- Autism, Asperger syndrome, pervasive developmental disorder not otherwise specified (PDD-NOS), childhood disintegrative disorder, and Rett syndrome, although usually only the first three conditions are considered part of the autism spectrum. These disorders are typically characterized by social deficits, communication difficulties, stereotyped or repetitive behaviors and interests, and in some cases, cognitive delays.

Autonomic Nervous System - is the part of the peripheral nervous system that acts as a control system, functioning largely below the level of consciousness, and controls visceral functions.[1] The ANS affects heart rate,digestion, respiratory rate, salivation, perspiration, pupillary dilation, micturition (urination), and sexual arousal. Most autonomous functions are involuntary but a number of ANS actions can work alongside some degree of conscious control. Everyday examples include

93

breathing, swallowing, and sexual arousal, and in some cases functions such as heart rate.

Chronic cerebrospinal venous insufficiency (CCSVI or CCVI) - a term developed by Italian researcher Paolo Zamboni in 2008 to describe compromised flow of blood in the veins draining the central nervous system

Chronic Lyme Disease – Having Lyme disease more than 4 weeks (as defined by the CDC) and suffering severe debilitating pain and illness for prolonged period of time.

Co-infections – Other pathogens that can be carried with the Lyme spirochete into the body simultaneously that can also cause damage and fatalities. Babesia, Bartonella, Ehrlichia, Colorado Tick Fever, Tick Relapsing Fever, Q Fever, Flavivirus, Rocky Mountain Spotted Fever, West Nile Virus, Tularemia, Micoplasma

Die Off – The affect of the body processing the toxic out put from bacteria, viruses, parasites, yeasts, etc in the body. It has been likened to a hangover, some more severe than others.

Herxheimer- is a reaction to endotoxins released by the death of harmful organisms within the body. In holistic medicine, it is sometimes referred to as a healing crisis, as it may coincide with recovery from an infectious disease, or a course of detoxification. It resembles bacterial sepsis. A byproduct of the spirochetes causes this reaction. Typically, the death of these bacteria and the associated release of neurotoxins occurs faster than the body can remove the substances. It usually manifests within a few hours of the first dose of any treatment to kill off the spirochete. It manifests as fever, chills, rigor, hypotension,headache, tachycardia, hyperventilation, vasodilation with flushing, myalgia (muscle pain), exacerbation of skin lesions and anxiety.

Lyme - an infectious disease carried by ticks caused by bacteria of genus Borrelia

Lymie – Any person suffering from Chronic Lyme Disease

Neurotoxin – The extrement product of the spirochete in its life cycle. Mass amounts are produced when the spirochete "die off". They are an extensive class of exogenous chemical neurological insults which can adversely affect function in both developing and mature nervous tissue.

Post Lyme Syndrome - Most medical experts believe that the lingering symptoms are the result of residual damage to tissues and the immune system that occurred during the infection. The body's "memory" of having chronic lyme disease

Sepsis - is a potentially deadly medical condition characterized by a whole-body inflammatory state caused by severe infection. It is caused by the immune system's response to a serious infection, most commonly bacteria, but also fungi, viruses, and parasites in theblood, urinary tract, lungs, skin, or other tissues.

Spirochete - bacteria, most of which have long, helically coiled (spiral-shaped) cells. The other most commonly known spirochete is syphilis

Resources

Lyme:

The One Minute Cure – Cavanaugh
The Yeast Connection – Crook
Detoxify or Die – Rogers
Beating Lyme Disease – Jernigan
Everyday Miracles by God's Design – Jernigan
Alkalize or Die - Theodore A. Baroody

Spiritual:

31 Days of Praise – Warren and Ruth Meyers
Streams in the Desert – Cowman
Jesus Calling – Sarah Young
Jesus Today – Sarah Young
Circle Maker – Mark Batterson
Drawing the Circle – Mark Batterson

Uplifting and Encouraging Reading:

Not a Fan – Kyle Idleman
I Am Second - Doug Bender, Sterrett, McCoy
Beautiful Outlaw – Eldridge
George Mueller – autobiography
Gathering Manna – Sue Fallin
Who is this Man? – John Ortberg
If You Want to Walk on Water You Have to Get Out of the Boat – John Ortberg
Fearless – Max Lucado
He Still Moves Stones – Max Lucado
The Boy Who Came Back From Heaven – Kevin and Alex Malarkey

Heaven is for Real – Todd Burpo
90 Minutes in Heaven – Don Piper
In a Pit with a Lion on a Snowy Day – Mark Batterson

Online:

https://www.facebook.com/justlivinglikethiswithLYME

http://justlivinglikethiswithlyme.com/

http://pinterest.com/jpfairbairn/just-living-like-this-with-lyme/

http://www.zazzle.com/justlivinglyme

www.lymeresearchalliance.org

Hansa Center for Optimum Health - http://hansacenter.com/

www.mercola.com

http://www.youngliving.com

www.bachflower.com

www.ccsvi.org

Lyme Search Engine, by Google - http://www.tiredoflyme.com/

https://sites.google.com/site/lymediseasemapproject/home

About the Author

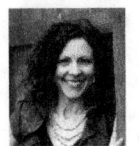

I am a 43 year old married, mother of 2. I discovered I had Lyme disease about 2012, after struggling most of 2011 with severe crashes and health crisis. I apparently had the slow workings of Lyme for over a decade because I gave everything I had to both my kids in the womb. They had been sick since birth and we had no idea what was going on with them. It has been a hard road, one that almost took my life as I hovered under 85 lbs, but it is one that has taught us all great life lessons and strengthened our faith.

As we were climbing out of our Lyme pit in 2013, I realized that God was compelling me to share my journey and give others who suffer a MEASURE OF HOPE.

In my previous life, I was a marketing and communications executive and then a work-from-home and stay-at-home mom. I have now become a PhD in health, healing, living right and all things Lyme. My passion is to see people embrace God's love and faithfulness by providing HOPE for their journey to healing. I love talking about health and healing to anyone who will listen. I adore my kids and how God has used our hardships to grow them into amazing young people with character and perseverance.

softcover book - http://www.amazon.com/author/janicefairbairn
Facebook - https://www.facebook.com/justlivinglikethiswithLYME
Blog - http://justlivinglikethiswithlyme.com/my-blog/
Twitter - https://twitter.com/lymeevangelist
Pintrest - http://www.pinterest.com/jpfairbairn/just-living-like-this-with-lyme/
YouTube - https://www.youtube.com/channel/UCul1VGlVLd6L0IjDwyPCOXg
Tumblr - http://janicelymeevangelist.tumblr.com/
ConnectPal - https://www.connectpal.com/janicefairbairn

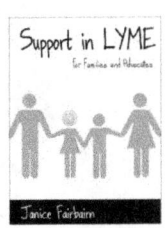

Support in LYME

For Families and Advocates

Also sold separately or as an ebook.

The LYME Diagnosis is devastating for many people who love a Lymie.

What you need to know to survive a loved one's trial with LYME. How to be a parent of a Lymie, how to be married to a Lymie, or how to be a friend and advocate to one. I cover all the bases on how to live through this with someone fighting to heal and live.

- What to do when you find out your spouse has Lyme
- How to cope with despair and discouragement along the way
- Learn how to be an advocate, fighting for your loved one to succeed
- Glean support and encouragement about how to be the parent of a Lymie child

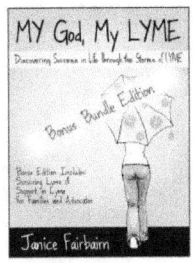

My God, My LYME

Discovering Success in Life
Through the Storms of LYME -
Bonus Bundle

Also sold separately or as an ebook.

Prepare for a Radical Battlefield. Includes Support in Lyme for Families and Advocates and Surviving Lyme.

Be inspired and encouraged by a true journey of faith through LYME. It's an amazing and real life success story. You can't help but be uplifted and gain strength from reading the story of one mom's compelling journey from the brink of death to healing and restoration for herself and her children from LYME.

Giving people the resources and HOPE they need for healing and how to live until they get there. Whether chronically ill with Lyme, already on your path to healing, or if you have conquered the mountain – this is for you.

- Discovering Success in Life out of the Storms of LYME.
- Be Inspired and Encouraged by this Journey of Faith
- Envision and Experience Whole Body Healing
- Prepare for a Radical Battlefield
- Get the Emotional and Spiritual Awakening You Desperately Need

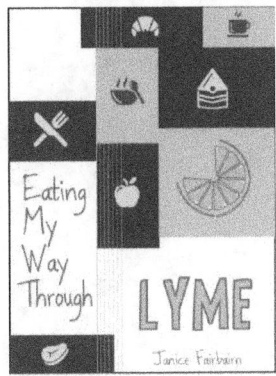

Don't Eat the Cardboard.

A Journey Eating My Way Through Lyme.

Available 2014 ebook.

www.selz.com

It is so hard to get well and get healthy at the same time.

I know going gluten free or dairy free just makes some of your head's spin. We've been gluten free, soy free and dairy free for almost 10 years now. These are adapted recipes and found recipes and combined recipes I've collected over the years to make our family happy and well fed. You don't have to do the research, you don't have to look for 5 years for a bread recipe that works or a pizza crust recipe your kids will eat – they are all in this collection. I am not a gormet cook, I'm just a mom who wanted to find recipes that worked without too much effort and that my family would enjoy. Your future in gluten free does not have to be bleak – you don't have to eat food that tastes like cardboard the rest of your life!!

https://justlivinglikethiswithlyme.selz.com/item/548b40d3b798720bbc12c742?mode=edit

Coming Soon!

Available for Pre-Sale on Amazon June 2016

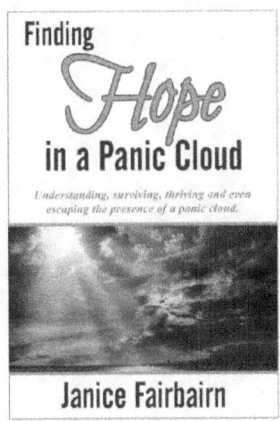

Is the Panic Cloud preventing you from living your life?

Do you feel that if you have faith you shouldn't feel scared or afraid?
Do you feel like if you have God in your life you should never panic?
Do you feel like your faith should keep you from having anxiety attacks
in overwhelming situations?

I used to think that I was failing somehow in my faith or that it wasn't
strong enough because I felt panic within life's circumstances that were
beyond my control. I felt as if I could not breathe at times and that I was
destined to live miserable and afraid in a giant Panic Cloud. Sometimes
the weight of our trials are a Panic Cloud that envelop and follow you
around choking your faith and ability to live. You don't have to feel that
way anymore.

There is HOPE.